OMERE
Speaks

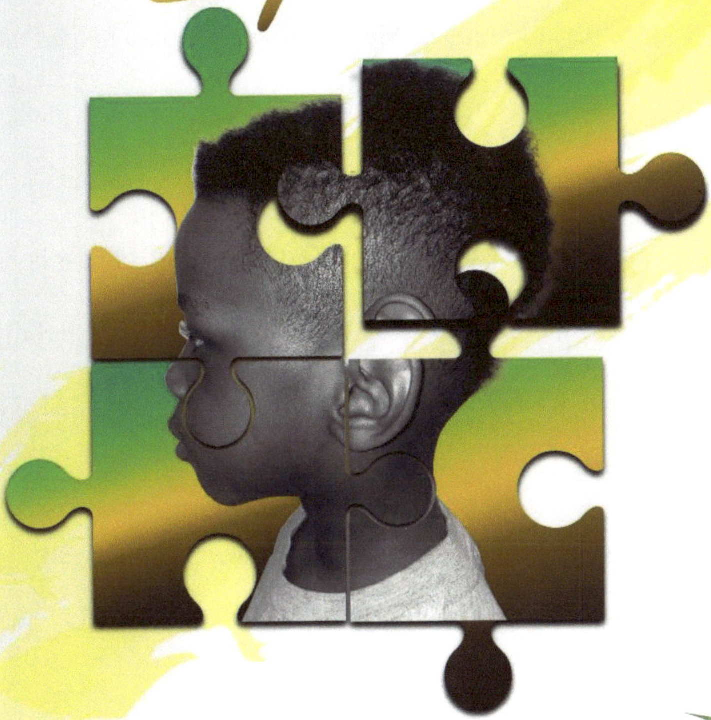

Acknowledgments

I would like to acknowledge and give my warmest thanks to all the people who helped Omere through this journey. The Charles and Brown family, Shillian Foreman, Maria Valladares, who helped us raise him. Our extended family, my W.O.L.F pack, "We Only Love Family" who always lifted me up and held me accountable. To the entire Hamaspik, Bravehood, ICLC and Tri-County Care staff and my loyal friends who continue to keep me grounded. To my loving sons Stephen and Omere, my two most precious kings, my reasons for being. Finally, to Omario, who kept his promise to me to be there for us, thank you.

Prologue

It was mid-afternoon on September 14, 2018, and we were waiting for Omere to undergo another set of examinations. Omario and I already knew the answer. However, we wanted confirmation that Omere was autistic. Honestly, we didn't care about the diagnosis but more so about the treatment plan and the required level and care that our 18-month-old son would need. Caring for a child with special needs was a new world for us. We had no idea what would be in store for our family, and how understanding the truth would change our lives. Omere was getting impatient, as most toddlers would, but since he couldn't vocalize what he needed to say, spinning around in circles was the

only way he calmed himself.

We're Pregnant

"I think you're pregnant. When was the last time you saw your period?". These were the exact words of my husband. I was a bit taken back because we've been through so much. My husband and I at the time were considering separation. However, with some counseling from his mom we made the decision to save our marriage. I eventually took a pregnancy test and anxiously waited for the results. This was the longest three minutes ever. Seeing the word "pregnant" shocked me. There was a 17-year gap between my soon to be child and my oldest son and I was not prepared for it.

Earlier on in our relationship, I was very adamant about not having more children. However, as our relationship grew, my feelings towards having another child began to change. I trusted my husband when he said he would always be there for our children, and he assured me that he would keep his word. My skepticism was due to my previous relationship and what I had endured while I was pregnant at the time. The lack of a consistent partner, the infidelity which subsequently led to me having to raise a child on my own. This wasn't an experience I wanted to relive. I just knew I did not want this to happen a second time around especially since we've had a tough year of marriage and now, having to decide on having a family together. It was a lot but I was determined to continue with this

pregnancy and so we decided to be the best parents
we could be.

My pregnancy was a challenging one. I was high-
risk because of my previous health conditions, and I
was almost forty. My OBGYN Physician was
concerned about my health, so she encouraged me
to join her pregnancy group which was for first time
moms, and moms who had a huge age gap in
between their children. She believed that being a
part of this group would reduce some of the stress I
was having.

Being a part of this group was very rewarding for
me. I was only twenty-one when I had my first baby
and I don't think anyone was taught how to be a
mom, and the resources at the time were limited.
During these group meetings, all the moms were

able to share their experiences. I felt so much support during these sessions. My Physician was right, it was a stress reliever knowing that I was not alone in this.

Another form of support I received from the group was getting a doula. She gave me all the necessary information I needed to get through delivery, and I was so grateful for this.

Unexpected Delivery

When I entered my third trimester, I was deemed a high-risk patient. I was required to be at the hospital once a week to ensure that everything was going well. After one of my visits, I received a phone call from the nurse who stated that my doctor wanted me to come back to the hospital. After reviewing my chart, the doctor noticed my son's heart rate was constantly dropping. She did not go into too many details but said that I urgently needed to be there and there was a possibility I would have to spend the night. My heart sank and I was so nervous. All I could think about was if my baby was okay. I quickly got my hospital bag and headed there.

After being monitored at the hospital for over six hours, a doctor finally saw me and made me aware that he would have to perform an emergency cesarean due to our son's heartbeat constantly going up and down. "Why was all of this happening?" "Was it something I did wrong?" "Was I not being a good mother to my child?" "Was this my punishment because I was against having another child?" All these doubts were racing through my head. I fought back the tears because I didn't want my stress level to contribute to what was already happening.

My husband finally arrived at the hospital with my best friend, Shelly. They were both giving me words of encouragement which kept me calm and helped me through. My doula called to check in on me and advised me that I could always get a second option and to contact my regular OB doctor.

My doctor finally called back after contacting him. He informed me that the hospital insisted on performing an emergency C-section. They were concerned about whether it would be successful since my platelets were low and I had underlying scar tissue from previous surgeries. He advised me not to agree to any procedure until he arrived so he could discuss my medical history with the on-site physician and formulate a plan for the baby and I. I vividly remember that it was 4:30 am, and my doctor advised me they could no longer wait for my platelets to increase. The surgery was to happen now. They had a specialist on-site in case of an emergency, along with blood for us. I remember being taken back into the operating room with my husband by my side. Having him there reassured me that everything would be okay. He constantly made me aware of how good I was doing, and that our baby would be okay. The surgery began, and baby Omere was born weighing 5lbs 2ozs. I didn't get a chance to hold him because the doctor immediately rushed him to the NICU to be monitored. Moments after, the nurse escorted my husband out of the operating room. I felt my body getting cold, and I was shaking. The doctor stated that it was due to all the blood I lost and that I would receive a blood transfusion. I began to say a silent prayer asking God to provide my husband with the strength he will need to take care of our son, and to allow me to hold our son before my time on this earth ends.

Welcome Home

A week passed since I gave birth to our prince. My anxiety was getting the best of me because I wanted him to come home with me. I was released from the hospital a week after delivery. However, due to Omere having jaundice, he was kept for an additional fifteen days. Those days felt like an entity. When I was finally able to take him home, it was such a rainy day I thought it was God's way of showing that he was here and that our prince was blessed. Being a new mom after so many years was a bit overwhelming, but I enjoyed every second of it. I grew so much and learned a lot more about motherhood this time around.

Omere was the toddler who slept during the day and stayed up at night. My husband worked overnight at the time, so it was just Omere and I which gave us an incredible bond. For the first two weeks of his birth, I couldn't have those bonding moments, so I cherished them as much as I possibly could and watched him grow. My life felt completed. I had a healthy baby boy, and although it was a seventeen-year gap between my oldest and Omere, I took pride in being present for both my boys.

Omere had the most prominent personality. When I spoke to him or played with him, he always had this intense look on his face as if he knew what I was saying. I asked him questions and allowed him time to respond whether it was with a giggle or a coo, it was so heartwarming.

As time passed, I noticed that he would not respond when I said his name. He wasn't crawling, sitting up, or walking like a "normal" baby would do and that scared me a bit. I knew from experience that he should've reached certain milestones. However, I was reassured by my mom that all children develop and grow differently, and that he is doing things at his own pace. She also told me that I was overthinking things so I let that thought go for a bit, but I couldn't help obsessing over ensuring that he reached these milestones based on the standards timetable.

Mama's Daycare

I am a strong believer that God puts people in our lives for a reason. Being back to work a month after giving birth was hard. It was not always easy to have a work and home life balance. Luckily, this is when I met my amazing mentor. She introduced me to a mentorship program that allowed me to envision myself more than just an employee. My vision was to become an entrepreneur, and one of my business ideas was to own a daycare. I even had a name in mind, and it was called "Mama's Daycare". At that time, I didn't know that I was manifesting Omere's new home away from home. Omere from two months of age spent his mornings with my eldest son's grandmother. This arrangement only lasted for a few months when she became ill, so it was time to place Omere into daycare.

While shopping for groceries one day, I came across a daycare called Mama's Daycare. My first thought was, is this a sign? Is this faith? How ironic this Daycare really exists. I immediately knew this was the place Omere needed to be. We stopped by the daycare the same day and filed out the necessary paperwork for him to attend there the following week. The very next day we were called in for a tour and to meet the owner 'Mama' and Omere's new teacher.

When we got to the Daycare, we felt welcomed and at home. This was the feeling I needed. There were learning charts on the wall, each child had their own cubby, and it was so clean. There were about fifteen children, and they were all separated by age and special needs. They all looked so well nurtured and taken care of. We knew he would've been in great hands.

Seven months into Omere attending Mama's daycare the owner wanted to speak with us about how well he was doing since he started attending there. Omere was such an easy-going baby, so we expected this of him. What we didn't expect was her concerns about him having autism. Her reason for this was due to her having raised and taught other children who had autism, she began to explain that she noticed some delay in his speech and fine motor skills. This is one of the hardest things any parent wants to hear. We all expect our baby to do great and to excel at everything they do, even as young as he was. The only thing I could've done in that moment was break down and cry. She saw our concerns and reassured us that every child develops differently and in their own time. Also, not because he isn't communicating or socially interacting as other children do, doesn't mean that he is not on the spectrum. She said that if he was delayed, he could receive the necessary resources to aid in his development.

Testing

Omere's 18-month checkup, this was so nerve wrecking. We had so many questions for the doctor regarding our baby's delays, not just speech but also his attention span. He was not responding when we called his name. He avoided all eye contact. The way he ate was not normal for an 18-month-old. This was finally the day we got to speak to a professional to have all these questions answered. Can Omere walk up and down a flight of stairs? Can he identify his shapes and colors? Can he grip pencils? Most importantly, can he speak? These were some of the screening questions that we had to answer. Honestly, who would've known that our toddler would have to undergo this type of intense screening. I never thought he would've had to express himself throughout all of this.

Omere became frustrated. He didn't understand why he had to do these things. When he got to this point, the only thing that kept him calm was to spin around in circles. My initial reaction was to tell him to stop spinning. I just didn't understand why he did this, and I knew in my heart that this was not a normal way of coping. This made him extremely sad. In his mind, this was the only way he knew how to stay calm. The observer also told him that him doing this could cause him and others pain. I noticed how upset he was becoming so I found a way to distract him. I gave him a task to complete. A task to organize toys by shape and color. It seemed to work for the most part. When he was all done, I encouraged him by cheering him on "Yay Omere! You did it!" And gave him a hi five.

Finally, after the tests were completed, Omere was diagnosed with autism spectrum disorder. We were both confused. We didn't know what to think. The observer noticed so she began to explain what autism spectrum disorder (ASD) was. It is a neurological and developmental disorder that affects how people learn, interact and communicate with others. Although autism can be diagnosed at any age, it is described as a developmental disorder because symptoms generally appear in the first two years of life. I was devastated. All I could think was why does it have to be my son? What is going to happen to him in the future? There were just so many questions I asked myself. I immediately had

to pull myself together. This was just one hurdle we

got to jump over together. I had to think of the

positives, our baby will now get the professional

help he needs to get through this.

Welcome To Hamaspik

After getting Omere's diagnosis, it was not easy finding the necessary resources to get him on track. I honestly thought I was going to have a meltdown. One day I expressed my frustration with my former administrative assistant, and she asked me if I've ever heard of Hamaspik. She mentioned that Hamaspik's mission is that every person, with their abilities and disabilities are unique. She was a case manager there and connected me to an intake coordinator so Omere can receive treatment. I felt like a huge weight was lifted off my shoulders. I was so relieved and was finally at peace. I didn't think we would've found a great program, but it all worked out.

The intake coordinator called me later that afternoon to schedule an appointment for us to come to their office, so Omere could be examined by one of their specialists. On the day of the appointment, we were taken to a conference room filled with sensory toys. A three-step staircase was to our immediate right. There was a coffee station, a sink, and a playpen. We were left in the room and two men came in right after to begin the assessment. I was nervous. All I could think about was what are these men going to say about to say about my son. Omere enjoyed the assessment. He didn't engage with the two men or make any eye contact. They said it was okay and wanted to see how he reacted when they entered the room. They asked us questions like when Omere began to walk; whether he responded to his name; how well he played with

other children, and whether he had any outbursts.

Let's Talk Therapy

Omere had an amazing therapist. Reminiscing with her in everything we've been through, this is what she said. "I was fortunate enough to be Omere's speech therapist and to have worked with him over his final school year. When I first met Omere, I was immediately shocked by his charm and sweetness. Whether in the classroom or during therapy sessions, he was always enthusiastic, motivated, and eager to be a "helper" whenever possible. Omere was a true gentleman, even at his tender age. I had never met a student who would prefer to say "I would like" rather than "I want" when requesting something. Though one of Omere's most endearing qualities were his passion for learning, it was just undeniable. He was one of my only students who chose reading over games as the target activity when given the opportunity. While understanding his speech was often a challenge, his genuine desire to grow and to progress shone through every moment. Additionally, what struck me was how incredibly self-aware he was and how this connectedness could be felt despite any articulatory or phonological obstacles. Omere is truly a remarkable young man."

"While I shared so many beautiful experiences with Omere as his speech therapist, one particularly noteworthy moment left quite an impression on me. I arrived at Omere's classroom one afternoon, and the teacher informed me that he had a reasonably challenging day due to unforeseen changes in their daily schedule. As Omere is a person who loves comfort and finds excellent security in consistency and routine, it did not surprise me that he had a horrible reaction to a change in an unexpected plan. After speaking with his mother, I understood Omere's distress tolerance and ability to process frustration during those problematic instances. Though, as mindful as I attempted to be, there was an additional, last-minute change in plans that proved to be just too overwhelming for Omere at this point. I inadvertently interrupted his snack time to carry out an activity rather than waiting for the snack to be concluded. At that point, I could see that Omere was becoming quite emotional and threw his head in his hands and laid down on the table, unable to respond to any questions. While this was certainly not what I had planned for our therapy session, it provided a unique and invaluable opportunity for myself and Omere."

"I utilized calming breath techniques, emotional co-regulation, and simple visual support. We created an environment where he could indicate his feelings and apply an alternative form of communication when verbal expressions were inaccessible. I was reminded that day as a therapist how essential it was to meet a student where they were in the moment rather than where we might feel they "should" be. I also sincerely believed that sessions like this one, wherein Omere was confronted with an unexpected change or a disappointment, were some of the most important. He only continued to grow throughout the school year, and became more and more adept at applying strategies to work through a problem rather than merely shutting down. These lessons were particularly crucial for students like Omere, who tend to be perfectionists. He was always diligent and tirelessly worked, even during some of the most tedious elements of speech therapy (e.g., sound errors). Though, he was also very hard on himself if things didn't work out exactly as he had imagined or if he felt he didn't meet an expectation. I provided opportunities for Omere to reckon with making mistakes. I also created a more compassionate internal monologue simultaneously, which were some of the most challenging and rewarding moments we shared."

Hearing Omere's teacher speak about his development gave me some ease. I knew he was progressing rapidly. However, I was also concerned that he was still lacking the basic skills he needed when it came to expressing himself. I honestly didn't know how to help him with this issue or where to even begin. I didn't have much patience when it came to being able to communicate with him, and I often blamed myself when I felt like he wasn't progressing. Still, I knew he would be able to find his way of expressing himself, and he always did it with a smile on his face. That helped me to do my best because I knew how much he needed me to be there for him.

Respite to the Rescue

Having a respite provider was so vital to Omere's growth. We had gone through three Health Aids, and each one was worse than the other. It was during the peak of the COVID pandemic where finding a caregiver was extremely difficult. All public schools were closed, and only essential workers were permitted to be out in public. It was a miracle that we even received a great provider. Maria was like a breath of fresh air. She made my transition back to work so smooth. She was attentive to Omere. She was patient and kind to him. The company she worked for had a system where she had to log everything she did for him via

Zoom. This wasn't always easy for her since she was not technologically savvy. Nevertheless, she overcame all the challenges thrown at her to ensure that all of Omere's needs were met.

Despite having an amazing caregiver Omere was faced with a few health scares. He was diagnosed with asthma. Every time we received a call from his school, we were terrified something was wrong. Those moments before picking up those calls felt like my heart was going to fall to the floor. We all know the feeling.

Also, during the pandemic Omere tested positive for COVD 19. This was a complete nightmare. Knowing the amount of people who died daily from this disease, put so much fear in us. For fourteen days, Omere fought for his life. He was constantly on his nebulizer to help with his breathing, the coughing and wheezing were never-ending, his fever was 102, and all we could've done was to keep faith that our son would survive this battle.

Autism as it relates to asthma or any other type of ailment, is a high tolerance or threshold for pain and discomfort. He doesn't usually express these things because he can't entirely process and explain his feelings, which as you can imagine, is a frustrating place to be. The most fantastic part about Omere is his upbeat personality. While we were in full panic mode, his calm demeanor was and is always quite remarkable. Seeing how joyful and optimistic he was, was the strength we needed to keep pushing through each trial.

Speak Up

While we were connected to Hamaspik, they led us to therapy to help Omere with his development. The process was challenging because everything was new to us. We needed to learn sign language to communicate since speaking was tough for Omere. Although he understood us, he had a really hard time being able to speak and communicate how he was feeling. Omere received part time therapy from 18 months to the age of 3. Once he reached the age of five he attended an integrated school.

During one of his therapy sessions, I remember they were teaching him 3 to 5 syllables. His teacher would always remind him to answer with a "say yes or no," she repeated the question, and he repeated 'yes, I can." His teacher was overjoyed and always had a massive smile on her face every time he hit a milestone. Meanwhile, I stood in the background with tears in my eyes because my son could now speak with clarity on what he could understand. He was now able to articulate his feelings with his therapist in 3 to 5 syllables. Before therapy, he would point to what he wanted, or he would take our hand and lead us to things he needed, or sometimes got frustrated and threw a tantrum when we were not able to understand. So, to have witnessed my son articulating himself was so just so amazing.

Graduation Day

Looking back at the past three years, a lot of things were brought into perspective. I witnessed our son overcome every obstacle life threw his way and I was so grateful at how strong and determined he was. Seeing him standing in front of a room filled with over one hundred people to accept his diploma was a full-circle moment. I remembered his father's words when we finally confirmed that we were pregnant.

He said, "someone once said you can plan a pretty picnic, but you can't predict the weather." Well, from that moment on, the weather has been beautiful. Sure, there were a lot of rainy days, but with Omere, it always felt sunny. He has such a vibrant articulate soul and is truly a gift from God himself. We couldn't imagine our lives would be altered in such an excellent way as this. Think about anything you love and desire the most, well, this is incomparable. It's a different kind of love that all parents experience. That indescribable feeling of joy overwhelms you whenever you look into their eyes. Each moment you want to hold on to forever, but can't as another soon replace it.

When I heard the doctor say, "baby out," I knew our lives would have never been the same. Omere has come a long way and honestly, we couldn't have done it alone. We thank the doctors who delivered him to his amazing respite provider, fairy Godmother Maria. Every day I think about our son and the strides he has made despite what he's going

through, tears fill my eyes, and I only have God to

thank for this.

Meet Omere

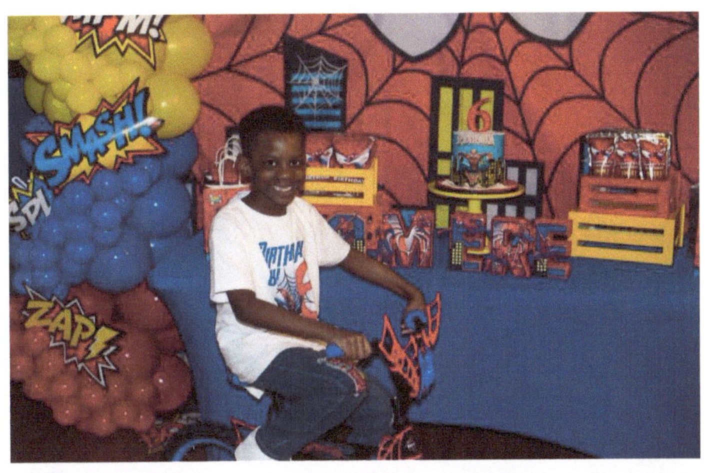

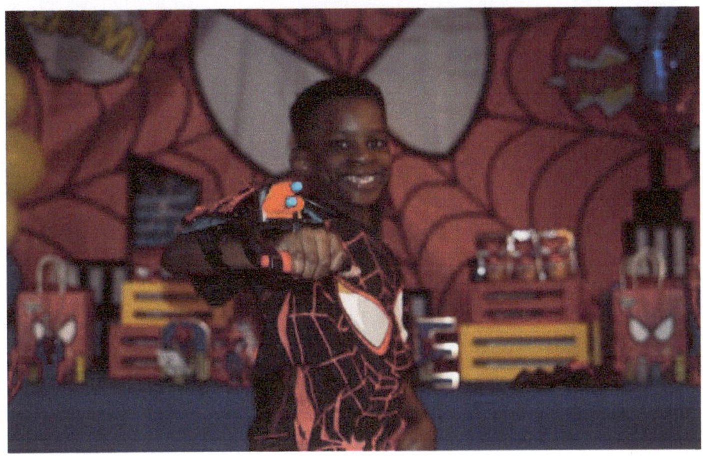

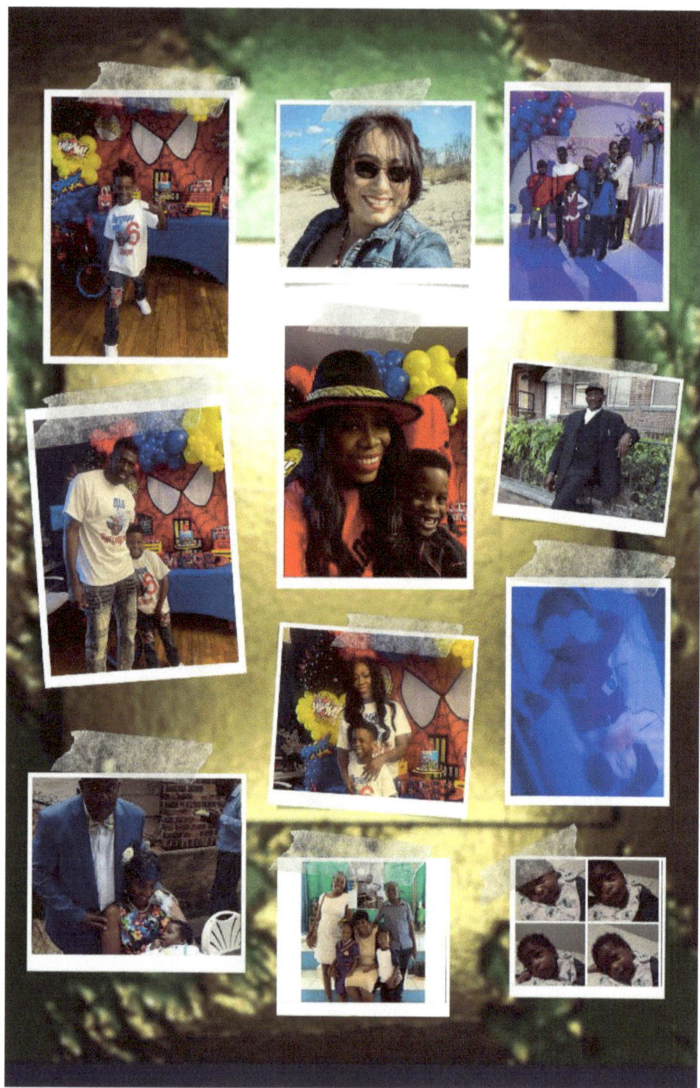

About The Author

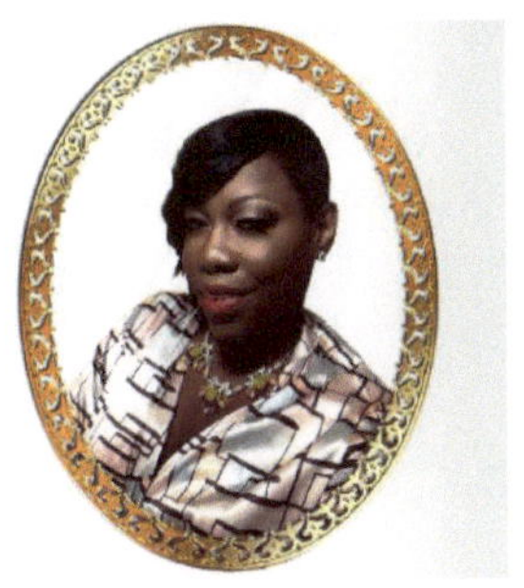

Nicole Jones was born in Jamaica and now reside in New York. She is a first-time author who wanted to share her journey. Prior to writing *Omere Speaks*, she's worked with hundreds of small and mid-sized businesses including the City of New York and Women on the Rise. Other services include Minority Certification Business Development and Branding Web design business credit. She has over 15 years of management and executive experience. She's currently obtaining her Bachelor of Arts and Master's degree at Monroe College.